THE ENERGY CODE: ACTIVATE CHAKRA HEALING AND ELEVATE YOUR LIFE

UNLOCK YOUR INNER POWER, BALANCE YOUR CHAKRAS, AND MANIFEST A VIBRANT, HIGH-ENERGY LIFE

EDELINE YU

Contents

Foreword   *v*

Preface   *vii*

Acknowledgements   *ix*

1. Content   1

2. Chapter 1: Understanding The Energy Code   4

3. Chapter 2: The Root Chakra – Foundation Of Stability   8

4. Chapter 3: The Sacral Chakra – Unlocking Creativity And   16
   Passion

5. Chapter 4: The Solar Plexus Chakra – Awakening Personal Power 24

6. Chapter 5: The Heart Chakra – The Power Of Love And   32
   Compassion

7. Chapter 6: The Throat Chakra – Expressing Your Truth   40

8. Chapter 7: The Third Eye Chakra – Activating Inner Wisdom   47

9. Chapter 8: The Crown Chakra – Connecting To Higher   56
   Consciousness

10. Chapter 9: The Energy Code In Daily Life   64

11. Chapter 10: Advanced Energy Mastery Practices   73

Foreword

I have been teaching chakra and energy meditation for quite some time and I think it's time for me to write a book to share the knowledge and the daily practical routines for benefits of others. My desire to help people are strong enough that propel me to venture into body and mind healing lanscape by using Reiki, energy management and meditation. Besides I am also providing life coaching to my clients in order to helps them to see clearer in their life direction and to face life challenges, from spiritual point of view.

Energy management is very important if one's wanted to sail smoothly in his or her life journey, regardless of any circumstances along the life. You never know what life will throw at you but they only things is to get ready yourself internally by mastering your own energy via chakra energy system.

Chakra energy system has been exist for thousands of years and it's only getting attention from people all over the world because that's the foundation of humand life energy. Via quanthum physics, it has been proven that human body is a complicated body consist of different frequency vibration, that makes up all the different organs and parts of the body, your thoughts, your emotion also an energy which can affect your overall body's energy state.

I hope you will find this book helpful in knowing fundamental principles of chakra system and energy world.

Thank you.

Preface

Energy is the foundation of everything we experience—our thoughts, emotions, physical well-being, and even our ability to manifest the life we desire. When our energy flows harmoniously, we feel vibrant, confident, and deeply connected to ourselves and the world around us. But when this flow is blocked or imbalanced, we may struggle with anxiety, fatigue, self-doubt, or a sense of being stuck in life.

I wrote "**The Energy Code**" to guide you on a journey of self-discovery, healing, and transformation through the power of the chakra system. This book is not just about theory; it's a practical roadmap to help you activate your chakras, clear energy blockages, and elevate your life to its highest potential.

In the pages ahead, we will explore:

- How energy works and why balancing your chakras is essential for overall well-being
- Techniques to ground yourself and create a strong energetic foundation through the Root Chakra
- Ways to unlock creativity, passion, and emotional flow with the Sacral Chakra
- How to build confidence and personal power through the Solar Plexus Chakra
- The key to opening your heart and experiencing deeper love and compassion with the Heart Chakra
- Tools for authentic self-expression and clear communication using the Throat Chakra
- Practices to sharpen intuition and inner wisdom by activating the Third Eye Chakra
- Methods to connect with your higher self and experience spiritual expansion through the Crown Chakra

But this book is not just about knowledge—it's about transformation. Each chapter will provide you with meditation techniques, energy exercises, and daily rituals that will help you integrate these practices into your everyday life. By the end of this journey, you'll have the tools to align your energy, awaken your full potential, and step into a life of clarity, joy, and purpose.

It's time to activate your Energy Code and embark on a path of profound healing and empowerment.

Are you ready? Let's begin.

Edeline Yu

Your Personal Chakra Energy Healing Mentor/Coach

Acknowledgements

Thank you to those we have inspired me and initiated me into the energy world that kickstart my own spiritiual growing journey.

Special deepest thanks to Beth, my yoga teacher who opened a door to me to step into the world of spirituality. My sincere thanks to William Lee Rand, my Reiki master who have inspired me to move forward based on my own soul path. Lastly thanks to Jusin, Jasper and Zoey for being my have been supporting me and teached me a lot about parenting with spirituality.

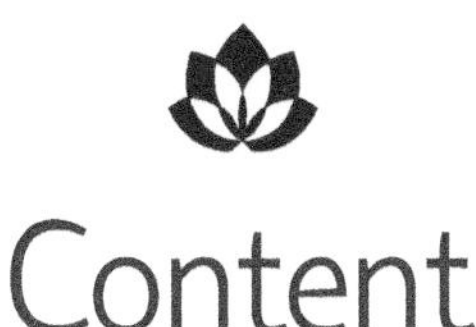

CHAPTER ONE

Content

Chapter 1: Understanding the Energy Code

- The science and spirituality of energy
- What are chakras and why they matter
- How energy flow shapes your physical, emotional, and spiritual well-being

Chapter 2: The Root Chakra – Foundation of Stability

- Healing fears, insecurities, and survival instincts
- Grounding techniques for stability and security
- Daily practices to strengthen your foundation

Chapter 3: The Sacral Chakra – Unlocking Creativity and Passion

- Emotional flow and creative expression
- Healing past emotional wounds
- Activating passion, pleasure, and joyful living

Chapter 4: The Solar Plexus Chakra – Awakening Personal Power

- Overcoming self-doubt and fear
- Boosting confidence and motivation
- Manifesting goals through empowered action

Chapter 5: The Heart Chakra – The Power of Love and Compassion

- Healing heart wounds and past traumas
- Cultivating self-love and deep relationships
- Practices for expanding love and gratitude

Chapter 6: The Throat Chakra – Expressing Your Truth

- Removing energetic blocks in communication
- Speaking with authenticity and clarity
- The power of affirmations and sound healing

Chapter 7: The Third Eye Chakra – Activating Inner Wisdom

- Strengthening intuition and insight
- Clearing mental fog and overthinking
- Meditation techniques for inner vision

Chapter 8: The Crown Chakra – Connecting to Higher Consciousness

- Expanding spiritual awareness
- Living in alignment with your higher self
- The role of meditation and energy transmission

Chapter 9: The Energy Code in Daily Life

- Aligning chakras with daily habits
- Creating a high-frequency lifestyle
- Chakra self-check practices

Chapter 10: Advanced Energy Mastery Practices

- Deepening your connection with energy work
- Combining breathwork, visualization, and movement
- Sustaining long-term energetic balance

Chapter 1: Understanding the Energy Code

The Science and Spirituality of Energy

Energy is the essence of life itself. It is the unseen force that animates our bodies, fuels our thoughts, and connects us to the universe. Across cultures and traditions, this life force has been given many names—*Prana* in Hinduism, *Qi (Chi)* in Chinese medicine, *Bioenergy* in modern science and *Mana* based on polinesia's culture.

From a scientific perspective, energy exists in everything. Our bodies function through electrical impulses, biochemical reactions, and electromagnetic fields. The heart generates an electrical charge, brain waves transmit signals, and every cell vibrates at a certain frequency. This energy can be measured, influenced, and balanced to improve overall well-being.

From a spiritual perspective, energy is the bridge between the physical and metaphysical. Ancient wisdom teaches that when our energy flows harmoniously, we experience health, clarity, and alignment with our true selves. When it is blocked, we may face emotional turmoil, illness, or a sense of being stuck in life.

The Energy Code is the key to understanding how energy flows within and around you. It is a system that integrates both the scientific and spiritual aspects of energy, helping you harness its power for healing, self-discovery, and transformation.

What Are Chakras and Why They Matter?

The chakra system is one of the most powerful energy models for understanding the human experience. The word "chakra" comes from Sanskrit and means "wheel" or "disc", referring to the spinning energy centers in the body that regulate physical, emotional, and spiritual health.

"There are seven main chakras, each associated with different aspects of life:"

Root Chakra (Muladhara) – Foundation, stability, survival
Sacral Chakra (Svadhisthana) – Creativity, emotions, pleasure
Solar Plexus Chakra (Manipura) – Confidence, personal power, motivation
Heart Chakra (Anahata) – Love, compassion, emotional healing
Throat Chakra (Vishuddha) – Communication, self-expression, truth
Third Eye Chakra (Ajna) – Intuition, wisdom, inner vision
Crown Chakra (Sahasrara) – Spiritual connection, higher consciousness

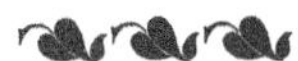

Each chakra is linked to specific organs, emotions, and mental states. When they are in balance, we feel centered, empowered, and in harmony. When blocked, they can lead to anxiety, fatigue, or physical discomfort.

Chakras are not just abstract concepts—they have a direct impact on your mood, relationships, decision-making, and even physical health. Understanding them is the first step in mastering your energy and unlocking your true potential.

How Energy Flow Shapes Your Physical, Emotional, and Spiritual Well-Being

Imagine your energy system as a river. When the water flows freely, everything is nourished, and life flourishes. But if there are blockages—like fallen trees or debris—the water stagnates, causing imbalance and disruption.

Your chakras operate the same way. When your energy flows smoothly:

✓ Physically – You feel energized, healthy, and free from chronic pain or illness.

✓ Emotionally – You are balanced, resilient, and able to process emotions with ease.

✓ Mentally – You have clarity, focus, and a strong sense of purpose.

✓ Spiritually – You feel connected to yourself, others, and the universe.

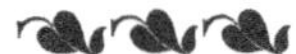

However, when energy gets blocked or imbalanced:

- You may feel exhausted, anxious, or overwhelmed.
- Unhealed traumas can surface as physical pain or emotional distress.
- Self-doubt, confusion, and lack of motivation can dominate your thoughts.

By learning to work with your chakras and clearing energy blockages, you can transform every area of your life. The tools in this book will help you do just that—through meditation, breathwork, movement, and daily rituals designed to activate your Energy Code and restore balance.

The Journey Ahead

In the following chapters, we will explore each chakra in depth, uncovering practical ways to balance and activate them. You will discover simple yet powerful techniques to:

- Increase your vitality and emotional resilience
- Overcome fear, stress, and limiting beliefs

- Tap into your creativity, confidence, and intuition
- Deepen your spiritual connection and live with purpose

Mastering your Energy Code is about more than just chakra healing—it's about aligning with your highest self and unlocking your fullest potential.

Are you ready to begin this transformational journey? Let's dive in.

Chapter 2: The Root Chakra – Foundation of Stability

Understanding the Root Chakra

The **Root Chakra (Muladhara)** is the first and foundational chakra in the energy system. Located at the *base of the spine*, it is associated with *stability, security, survival*, and *grounding*. The word Muladhara comes from Sanskrit, where Mula means "root" and Adhara means "support" or "foundation."

> *"This chakra governs our basic needs—food, shelter, safety, financial security, and emotional stability. When balanced, you feel safe, grounded, and confident in navigating life's challenges. When blocked or imbalanced, you may experience fear, insecurity, instability, or financial struggles."*

The Root Chakra is the foundation of the entire chakra system. If it is weak or unstable, energy cannot flow freely through the other chakras, affecting your physical health, emotional well-being, and spiritual growth.

- **Formation Period** : from birth to one year old
- **Location**: at the end of the vertebrae, at the perineum, including the legs and feet
- **Color** : Red
- **Element**: Earth
- **Nature of energy**: Yin
- **Sound**: LANG

Healing Fears, Insecurities, and Survival Instincts

Signs of an Imbalanced Root Chakra

A blocked or underactive Root Chakra may cause:

- Chronic anxiety, fear, or insecurity
- Feeling ungrounded or disconnected from reality
- Financial instability or struggles with abundance
- Lack of motivation and difficulty making decisions
- Low energy, fatigue, or lower back pain

An overactive Root Chakra can manifest as:

- Excessive materialism or obsession with security
- Fear of change and resistance to new experiences
- Aggressiveness or controlling behavior
- Hoarding tendencies or attachment to possessions

Healing the Root Chakra

The key to healing your Root Chakra is to address deep-seated fears and insecurities while cultivating a sense of safety and trust in life. Here are some healing approaches:

1. Acknowledge and Release Fear

- Write down your fears and insecurities. Ask yourself: Are these fears real, or are they based on past experiences and limiting beliefs?
- Practice self-affirmations such as:

> *"I am safe. I am secure. I trust life to support me."*

2. Reconnect with Your Body

- Since the Root Chakra is linked to physical survival, engaging in body-based practices helps restore balance.
- Try yoga, walking barefoot (earthing), or grounding meditation to reconnect with your body and the earth.

3. Heal Trauma and Inner Child Wounds

- Many Root Chakra imbalances stem from childhood experiences of instability or lack of safety.
- Inner child healing meditations and journaling can help release old fears and rebuild a sense of trust.

Grounding Techniques for Stability and Security

Grounding is essential for keeping the Root Chakra strong. When you are grounded, you feel centered, present, and connected to reality. Here are some powerful grounding techniques:

1. Grounding Meditation

Visualization: Imagine roots growing from the soles of your feet, extending deep into the earth. Feel the stability and nourishment from the earth's energy, anchoring you in the present moment.

2. Walking Barefoot (Earthing)

Walking barefoot on grass, sand, or soil connects your energy to the earth. This practice helps discharge excess energy, relieve stress, and strengthen your Root Chakra.

3. Root Chakra Affirmations

Repeat daily:

- "I am grounded and secure."
- "I trust the universe to support me."
- "I have everything I need."

4. Using Root Chakra Stones

Crystals like Red Jasper, Hematite, Smoky Quartz, and Black Tourmaline help absorb negative energy and enhance stability. Carry them in your pocket or place them near your bed.

5. *Eating Grounding Foods*

Nourish your Root Chakra with red and earthy foods like:

- Root vegetables (carrots, potatoes, beets)
- Red fruits (strawberries, cherries, apples)
- Proteins and whole grains for physical strength

Daily Practices to Strengthen Your Foundation

To keep your Root Chakra strong and balanced, incorporate these daily habits:

- **Morning Grounding Ritual** – Start your day by standing barefoot outside for a few minutes, breathing deeply, and visualizing yourself as strong and rooted like a tree.
- **Movement and Exercise** – Engage in physical activities like yoga, tai chi, or strength training to enhance body awareness and stability.
- **Financial and Emotional Stability Check-ins** – Take small, practical steps toward financial security and emotional well-being. This can include budgeting, planning, or setting clear boundaries in relationships.
- **Connect with Nature** – Spend time outdoors, go for walks, or practice mindful gardening. Nature naturally balances the Root Chakra.
- **Evening Gratitude Practice** – Before bed, write three things you are grateful for. Gratitude shifts your focus from fear to abundance.
- **Chakra Sound Healing** - Chanting the sacral mantra "LANG" or listening to singing bowl frequencies (396 Hz) can clear blockages.

Conclusion: Building a Strong Foundation for Growth

Balancing the Root Chakra is the *first step in activating your Energy Code.* It provides the stability, confidence, and security needed to thrive in all areas of life. When your foundation is strong, you can move forward with clarity, resilience, and trust in the universe.

> "*As you integrate these grounding practices, you'll notice a greater sense of peace, stability, and empowerment. Your fears will start to fade, and you'll feel more present and connected to yourself and the world.*"

Now that your foundation is set, we will explore the **Sacral Chakra**—the center of creativity, passion, and emotional flow. Let's dive in!

Chapter 3: The Sacral Chakra – Unlocking Creativity and Passion

Introduction: The Power of the Sacral Chakra

The Sacral Chakra (Svadhisthana) is the center of *creativity*, *passion*, *emotions*, and *pleasure*. Located just below the navel, in the lower abdomen.

> *"This chakra governs our ability to express ourselves freely, experience joy, and embrace intimacy. The word Svadhisthana means "one's own dwelling place", reminding us to reconnect with our true essence."*

When your Sacral Chakra is balanced, you feel emotionally fluid, inspired, and confident in your creative expression. You can embrace pleasure without guilt and cultivate deep, fulfilling relationships.

However, when blocked or imbalanced, you may struggle with:

- Emotional numbness or instability
- Creative blocks and lack of inspiration
- Fear of intimacy or difficulty forming deep connections
- Suppressed desires and guilt around pleasure
- Low libido or an excessive focus on sensual indulgence

In this chapter, we'll explore how to heal, activate, and fully harness the passionate, creative, and joyful energy of the Sacral Chakra.

- **Formation Period** : from 6 months to 2 years old
- **Location**: On the abdomen, between the navel and the buttocks, including the lower back, pelvis and sexual organs.
- **Color** : Orange
- **Element**: Water
- **Nature of energy**: Yin
- **Sound**: VANG

Emotional Flow and Creative Expression

The Sacral Chakra is deeply connected to our emotions and creative life force. It allows us to feel deeply, express ourselves freely, and embrace life's pleasures without fear or guilt.

Signs of a Blocked Emotional Flow

When emotional energy is suppressed or stagnant, it can manifest as:

- Emotional repression or fear of vulnerability
- Mood swings or excessive emotional reactions
- Creative blocks or feeling uninspired
- Self-doubt and lack of motivation

Restoring Emotional Balance

To unblock emotional flow, it's important to allow yourself to feel without judgment. Here's how:

1. **Emotional Journaling** – Write freely about your emotions, past wounds, and desires. Acknowledge your feelings without suppression.
2. **Express Through Art** – Painting, dancing, singing, or any creative outlet can release trapped emotions and awaken your creative energy.
3. **Water Therapy** – Since the Sacral Chakra is associated with water, activities like bathing, swimming, or listening to water sounds can help restore emotional balance.
4. **Dance and Movement** – Fluid body movements, especially hip-focused exercises like belly dancing or yoga, can release stagnant energy and increase your creative flow.

Healing Past Emotional Wounds

Many Sacral Chakra imbalances stem from *unresolved emotional wounds*—especially from childhood, past relationships, or societal conditioning around pleasure and self-expression.

Common Emotional Wounds Stored in the Sacral Chakra

- **Fear of rejection** – Holding back emotions due to past experiences of judgment or betrayal.
- **Shame around pleasure** – Feeling guilt or unworthiness when embracing joy, intimacy, or desires.
- **Heartbreak and loss** – Emotional pain from past relationships affecting the ability to connect deeply.
- **Fear of failure** – Suppressed creativity due to past experiences of criticism or self-doubt.

Healing Practices

Inner Child Healing

- Visualize yourself as a child and send love and reassurance to your younger self.
- Speak affirmations like: "I am free to feel and express myself fully."

Forgiveness Ritual

- Write a letter to someone (or yourself) who has hurt you.
- Express all your emotions, then burn or release the letter in water as a symbolic act of letting go.

Chakra Sound Healing

- Chanting the sacral mantra "VANG" or listening to singing bowl frequencies **(417 Hz)** can clear blockages.

Essential Oils for Emotional Release

- Orange, sandalwood, and ylang-ylang oils stimulate creativity, pleasure, and emotional healing.

Activating Passion, Pleasure, and Joyful Living

The Sacral Chakra is the seat of passion, sensuality, and pleasure. Activating it means giving yourself permission to experience joy fully, without guilt or fear.

Ways to Awaken Passion and Joy

1. Reignite Your Creative Spark

- Try something new—paint, write, cook, dance!
- Engage in hobbies that excite and inspire you.

2. Embrace Sensuality

- Sensuality is not just about intimacy—it's about fully experiencing life through the senses.
- Engage in activities that bring pleasure:

  - Eat vibrant, flavorful foods
- Listen to music that moves your soul
- Spend time in nature and appreciate beauty

3. Connect with Your Body

- Practice self-massage, yoga, or gentle stretching to awaken body awareness and self-love.
- Wear orange-colored clothing to stimulate the Sacral Chakra.

4. Affirmations for Joy and Creativity

- "I embrace pleasure and creativity without fear."
- "I allow my emotions to flow freely and fully."
- "I am passionate, joyful, and open to life's experiences."

Conclusion: Flowing Freely into a Creative, Passionate Life

A *balanced Sacral Chakra* allows you to:

- Express emotions freely and confidently
- Embrace creativity without fear of judgment
- Experience pleasure and passion in all areas of life
- Form deep, meaningful relationships

"*When your Sacral Chakra is activated, you will feel alive, inspired, and deeply connected to your emotions, desires, and creative essence.*"

In the next chapter, we will explore the **Solar Plexus Chakra**, the center of confidence, personal power, and motivation. Get ready to step into your full potential!

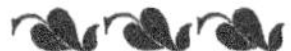

Chapter 4: The Solar Plexus Chakra – Awakening Personal Power

Introduction: The Power Within

The **Solar Plexus Chakra (Manipura)** is the center of personal power, confidence, and self-worth. Located in the upper abdomen, just above the navel.

> "*This chakra governs motivation, willpower, and the ability to take decisive action. The Sanskrit word Manipura means "city of jewels," symbolizing the radiant energy within you that fuels your strength and determination.*"

When the Solar Plexus Chakra is balanced, you feel:

- Confident in yourself and your decisions
- Motivated to take action toward your goals
- Capable of overcoming challenges with resilience
- In control of your emotions and personal boundaries

However, when blocked or imbalanced, you may experience:

- Self-doubt, low self-esteem, or fear of failure
- Lack of motivation and procrastination
- Feeling powerless or unable to make decisions
- Digestive issues or fatigue

In this chapter, we'll explore how to release fear, build self-confidence, and step into your full power through energy work, mindset shifts, and daily empowerment practices.

- **Formation Period** : from 18 months to 3 years old
- **Location**: The area above the navel, around the diaphragm,
- **Color** : Yellow
- **Element**: Fire
- **Nature of energy**: Yang
- **Sound**: RANG

Overcoming Self-Doubt and Fear

The Root of Self-Doubt

Self-doubt often stems from past conditioning, criticism, or fear of failure. It manifests as negative self-talk, hesitation, or feeling unworthy of success. To heal, we must shift our inner dialogue and reclaim our sense of personal power.

Signs of a Blocked Solar Plexus Chakra

- Difficulty standing up for yourself
- Seeking approval from others to feel validated
- Struggling to take action due to fear of failure
- Feeling powerless or out of control in situations

Healing and Strengthening Your Inner Power

1. Rewriting Your Inner Story

- Identify limiting beliefs (e.g., "I'm not good enough" or "I don't have what it takes").
- Replace them with empowering affirmations, such as:

  "I am strong, capable, and confident."

  "I trust myself to make the right decisions."

2. Facing Your Fears Head-On

- List your fears and challenge them by asking: "What's the worst that could happen? Is it really true?"
- Take small, courageous steps outside your comfort zone daily.

3. Breathwork for Confidence

- Try deep diaphragmatic breathing to activate the Solar Plexus Chakra and release tension.
- A powerful technique: Bhastrika (bellows breath) – rapid, forceful inhales and exhales through the nose to energize the body and mind.

Boosting Confidence and Motivation

When your Solar Plexus Chakra is open, you naturally radiate confidence, determination, and self-trust. You take inspired action without fear and remain resilient in the face of obstacles.

Daily Practices for Confidence

- **Power Posing**: Stand in a strong, expansive stance for two minutes each morning to activate feelings of strength and self-assurance.
- **Morning Visualization**: Close your eyes and visualize a bright yellow sun radiating at your solar plexus, filling you with confidence and motivation.
- **Chakra Sound Healing**: Chant "RANG", the Solar Plexus mantra, or listen to **528 Hz** frequency music to activate this energy center.

Movement and Core Activation:

- Yoga poses like Boat Pose, Warrior Pose, and Twists help energize this chakra.
- Engage in core-strengthening exercises like planks and crunches to activate your personal power.

Wearing Yellow: Incorporate yellow clothing or accessories to stimulate your confidence and self-worth.

Manifesting Goals Through Empowered Action

The Solar Plexus Chakra is the bridge between desire and manifestation. It gives you the drive and discipline to turn dreams into reality.

How to Take Aligned Action

1. Clarity is Power

- Define your goals with precision: What do you truly want? Why is it important?
- Write your intentions down to strengthen your focus.

2. Break It Down

- Divide big goals into small, actionable steps to avoid overwhelm.
- Set daily or weekly milestones to track progress.

3. Trust Your Decisions

- Stop second-guessing yourself. Take action even if you feel uncertain—confidence grows through experience.

4. Overcome Procrastination

- The 5-Second Rule: Count down from 5 to 1 and immediately take action to bypass hesitation.
- Practice accountability—share your goals with a friend or mentor.

5. Embody Your Future Self

- Ask yourself: How would the most confident, powerful version of me act today? Then, embody that energy.

Conclusion: Step Into Your Power

By balancing your Solar Plexus Chakra, you unlock your inner warrior—a version of yourself that is:

- Unstoppable in pursuing goals
- Fearless in making bold decisions
- Confident in personal worth and abilities
- Empowered to take control of life

> "*When you own your power, you become a conscious creator of your destiny. Let your inner fire burn brightly and guide you toward success.*"

In the next chapter, we will explore the **Heart Chakra**—the gateway to love, compassion, and deep emotional healing. Get ready to open your heart and connect on a soul level.

Chapter 5: The Heart Chakra – The Power of Love and Compassion

Introduction: The Gateway to Love

The **Heart Chakra (Anahata)** is the center of *love, compassion,* and *emotional connection.* Located at the center of the chest, it serves as a bridge between the lower chakras (physical and personal power) and the higher chakras (spiritual awareness and intuition).

> "*The Sanskrit word Anahata means "unstruck sound", symbolizing unconditional love that is limitless and pure.*"

When your Heart Chakra is open and balanced, you feel:

- Deep self-love and acceptance
- Compassion for others and the ability to forgive
- Harmonious and meaningful relationships
- Gratitude, joy, and emotional peace

When the Heart Chakra is blocked, you may experience:

- Emotional pain, resentment, or difficulty forgiving
- Fear of vulnerability or difficulty forming deep connections
- Feeling unworthy of love or seeking external validation

- Loneliness, isolation, or excessive dependence on others

In this chapter, we'll explore how to heal past emotional wounds, cultivate self-love, and expand the power of love and gratitude in your life.

- **Formation Period** : from 3 to 7 years old
- **Location**: The area on the center of the chest
- **Color** : Green
- **Element**: Air
- **Nature of energy**: Yang/Yin
- **Sound**: YANG

Healing Heart Wounds and Past Traumas

Many heart chakra blockages stem from past emotional pain, including heartbreak, betrayal, childhood wounds, or loss. When we hold onto these wounds, we close ourselves off from love and connection. Healing the Heart Chakra requires releasing old pain, practicing forgiveness, and reopening ourselves to love.

Signs of an Unhealed Heart Chakra

- Holding onto past resentment or heartbreak
- Fear of trusting others due to past betrayals
- Feeling emotionally numb or disconnected from love
- Difficulty in expressing or receiving love

Healing Practices for the Heart Chakra

1. Forgiveness Ritual

- Write a letter to someone who has hurt you (or to yourself) expressing everything you feel.
- You don't need to send it—burn it or tear it up as a symbolic release.
- Repeat the affirmation: "I release the past and open my heart to love."

2. Heart-Centered Meditation

- Close your eyes and visualize a green light glowing in your chest.
- With each breath, expand this energy and allow it to expand to the whole body.
- When breath out, imagine the out breath dissolve all the emotional pain.

3. Chakra Sound Healing

- Chant "YANG", the Heart Chakra mantra, to vibrate healing energy through your heart space.
- Listen to **639 Hz** frequencies for emotional healing and love expansion.

4. Crystal Therapy

- Wear or meditate with rose quartz (stone of unconditional love) or green aventurine (stone of emotional healing).

5. Letting Go Exercise

- Write down what emotional pain you are holding onto.
- Say out loud: "I lovingly release what no longer serves me."
- Tear up the paper and dispose of it with gratitude (burning it with fire will be good).

Cultivating Self-Love and Deep Relationships

Before we can truly love others, we must learn to love ourselves. Self-love is not about ego or selfishness—it is about respecting, accepting, and nurturing yourself fully.

Signs of Low Self-Love

- Negative self-talk or self-criticism
- Seeking external validation for worthiness
- Difficulty setting boundaries in relationships
- Feeling unworthy of love or affection

Self-Love Practices

Mirror Affirmations –

Stand in front of a mirror, look into your own eyes, and say:

- "I am worthy of love."
- "I deeply and completely love myself."
- "I accept myself as I am."

Heart-Opening Yoga Poses

– Practice poses that stretch the chest, such as:

- Cobra Pose
- Camel Pose
- Bridge Pose

Nurturing Yourself Daily

– Do things that bring you joy and relaxation:

- Take a warm bath with rose essential oil
- Spend time in nature, absorbing the beauty around you
- Write love letters to yourself about your strengths and beauty

Setting Healthy Boundaries

– Recognize that saying no to toxic relationships or energy-draining situations is an act of self-love.

Practices for Expanding Love and Gratitude

An open Heart Chakra allows you to radiate love, compassion, and gratitude effortlessly. The more love you give, the more you receive.

Daily Gratitude Practice

- Keep a gratitude journal and write three things you're grateful for every day.
- Before bed, place your hand over your heart and say:

  - *"I am grateful for the love in my life."*
  - *"My heart is open to giving and receiving love."*

Acts of Kindness

Perform one random act of kindness daily—it could be as simple as smiling at a stranger or giving a heartfelt compliment.
Express appreciation to the people in your life—call or message someone just to say you appreciate them.

Heart-Opening Visualization

- Sit quietly and visualize a golden light surrounding your heart, expanding outward like ripples in water, touching your loved ones and beyond.
- Imagine this light radiating across the world, filling it with love and compassion.

Conclusion: Living with an Open Heart

A balanced Heart Chakra allows you to:

- Love yourself unconditionally
- Forgive and release emotional pain
- Attract deep, meaningful relationships
- Feel a profound sense of gratitude and joy

> *"When your Heart Chakra is open, love flows effortlessly in your life. You become a magnet for compassion, connection, and deep fulfillment."*

In the next chapter, we'll explore **the Throat Chakra,** the center of authentic communication, self-expression, and truth. Get ready to speak your truth with clarity and confidence!

Chapter 6: The Throat Chakra – Expressing Your Truth

Introduction: The Voice of Your Soul

The **Throat Chakra (Vishuddha)** is the energy center of communication, truth, and self-expression. Located at the base of the throat, it governs how you speak, listen, and express your authentic self.

> "*The Sanskrit name Vishuddha means "pure" or "purification," signifying that speaking the truth is an act of cleansing and alignment.*"

When your Throat Chakra is open and balanced, you:

- Express yourself clearly and confidently
- Communicate with honesty and authenticity
- Feel heard and understood by others
- Listen deeply and speak with wisdom

However, when your Throat Chakra is blocked, you may experience:

- Fear of speaking up or expressing your opinions
- Difficulty finding the right words to communicate
- Tendency to suppress emotions or hold back thoughts

- Throat discomfort, tension, or frequent throat-related issues

In this chapter, we'll explore how to clear energetic blocks, speak with authenticity, and harness the power of affirmations and sound healing to strengthen your voice and truth.

- **Formation Period** : from 7 to 10 years old
- **Location**: The area on throat
- **Color** : Ocean Blue
- **Element**: Vibration/Ether
- **Nature of energy**: -
- **Sound**: HANG

Removing Energetic Blocks in Communication

The Throat Chakra can become blocked due to fear, past trauma, or societal conditioning. Many people suppress their truth out of fear of judgment, rejection, or conflict, leading to a lack of self-expression.

Signs of a Blocked Throat Chakra

? Holding back thoughts or feelings to avoid confrontation
? Feeling like your voice is not heard or valued
? Speaking too little or too much (e.g., over-explaining or being overly shy)
? Difficulty in public speaking or expressing emotions verbally

Healing Practices for the Throat Chakra

Journaling for Clarity

- Write freely about what you truly feel but have never expressed.
- Ask yourself: "What truths am I afraid to speak?"
- Practice writing letters to your younger self or to someone you need closure with.

Breathwork for Vocal Release

- Lion's Breath: Inhale deeply, then exhale forcefully with your tongue out, making a sound 'eh'. This helps clear stagnant energy from the throat.

Speaking Your Truth Exercise

- Stand in front of a mirror and say: "My voice matters. I speak my truth with confidence and ease."

- Practice saying NO when something doesn't align with your truth.

Release Judgment and Fear

• 43 •

- Accept that not everyone has to agree with you—your truth is valid.
- Let go of the fear of being "wrong" and embrace authentic self-expression.

Speaking with Authenticity and Clarity

True communication is not just about speaking—it's also about listening, understanding, and aligning your words with your inner truth. When you speak authentically, your words hold power, and people resonate with your message.

How to Cultivate Authentic Communication

Speak from the Heart:

- Before speaking, pause and ask: "Is this true? Is this necessary? Is this kind?"
- Avoid speaking from ego or fear—instead, let your words reflect your inner wisdom.

Practice Assertive Communication:

- Use "I" statements instead of blaming (e.g., "I feel unheard when..." instead of "You never listen").
- Express needs and boundaries clearly, without aggression or passivity.

Develop Active Listening:

- Truly listen without preparing your response while the other person is speaking.
- Make eye contact, nod, and acknowledge the speaker's emotions.

Slow Down and Speak with Intention:

- Take deep breaths before speaking to ground yourself.
- Use pauses to give your words weight and clarity.

The Power of Affirmations and Sound Healing

Affirmations for the Throat Chakra

""*My voice is powerful, and my words matter.*"
"*I express my truth with clarity and confidence.*"
"*I communicate openly and honestly.*"
"*I trust my inner voice and speak with courage.*""

Chanting and Mantras

Sound vibrations are deeply healing for the Throat Chakra.

- Chant "HANG" (the Throat Chakra mantra) for 3–5 minutes daily.
- Sing, hum, or recite poetry to activate the vocal cords.

Sound Frequency Healing

The Throat Chakra resonates with the **741 Hz** frequency, which:

- Clears toxins and negative energy from communication patterns
- Helps unlock self-expression and creativity
- Enhances clarity and openness in speech

Listen to 741 Hz music or use singing bowls tuned to this frequency for deep chakra healing.

Conclusion: Owning Your Voice

When your Throat Chakra is balanced, you:

- Speak with confidence, clarity, and authenticity
- Feel heard, valued, and respected
- Communicate your needs without fear
- Express emotions freely and honestly

Your voice is a gift—it has the power to heal, inspire, and create change. By speaking your truth, you step into your full authenticity and align with your highest self.

In the next chapter, we will explore the **Third Eye Chakra**, the center of intuition, wisdom, and inner guidance. Get ready to awaken your inner vision and deeper knowing!

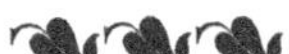

Chapter 7: The Third Eye Chakra – Activating Inner Wisdom

Introduction: Awakening Your Inner Vision

The **Third Eye Chakra (Ajna)** is the center of intuition, inner wisdom, and higher perception. Located between the eyebrows.

> *"This chakra governs our ability to see beyond the physical realm, access deeper insights, and trust our inner guidance."*

The Sanskrit word Ajna means "perception" or "command," reflecting its role in guiding us toward clarity, wisdom, and spiritual awareness.

When your Third Eye Chakra is open and balanced, you:

- Trust your intuition and inner knowing
- See life with clarity and deeper understanding
- Make aligned decisions with confidence
- Experience vivid dreams and heightened awareness

However, when the Third Eye Chakra is blocked, you may experience:

- Overthinking and mental fog
- Self-doubt and difficulty making decisions
- Feeling disconnected from your intuition

- A rigid, logical mindset that rejects spiritual insight

In this chapter, we'll explore how to strengthen intuition, clear mental fog, and activate your inner vision through meditation and energy practices.

- **Formation Period** : during teenager stage
- **Location**: The area on the center of the two eyebrow
- **Color** : Indigo
- **Element**: Light
- **Nature of energy**: Yang
- **Sound**: AUM

Strengthening Intuition and Insight

Intuition is our inner guidance system—a deep knowing that comes from within, beyond logic and reason. A strong Third Eye Chakra allows us to trust our instincts, see through illusions, and align with our highest wisdom.

Signs of a Weak Intuition

- Constantly seeking external validation for decisions
- Ignoring gut feelings and later regretting it
- Feeling lost or disconnected from life's purpose
- Overanalyzing situations instead of trusting inner knowing

Practices to Enhance Intuition

Journaling for Inner Guidance

- Every morning, write down any intuitive nudges or gut feelings you experienced the previous day.
- Reflect on how they turned out—over time, this builds trust in your intuition.

Decisive Action Practice

- For small daily choices (e.g., what to eat, where to go), pause and tune into your inner feeling before deciding.
- Ask yourself: "Does this feel right for me?" instead of overanalyzing.

Symbol Interpretation Exercise

- Pay attention to recurring symbols, dreams, and synchronicities—they are messages from your higher self.
- Keep a dream journal and write down symbols that appear often.

Strengthening Your Gut-Brain Connection

- Intuition is often felt in the gut (the "second brain").
- Eat clean, high-vibration foods to keep this connection strong.

Clearing Mental Fog and Overthinking

A blocked Third Eye Chakra often manifests as *overthinking, confusion,* or *lack of mental clarity.* When we are too caught up in logic, fears, or outside opinions, our ability to trust our inner wisdom becomes clouded.

Causes of Mental Fog & Overthinking

- Excessive screen time & digital overstimulation
- Relying only on rational thinking and ignoring intuition
- Unresolved fears creating mental clutter
- Lack of time in stillness or self-reflection

How to Clear the Mind for Clarity

Digital Detox

- Spend at least one hour a day without screens.
- Limit social media scrolling, which overloads the brain with information.

Nature Connection

- Go outside, breathe deeply, and observe without judgment.
- Walk barefoot on the earth to reset your energy field.

Breathwork for Mental Clarity

- Practice alternate nostril breathing (Nadi Shodhana) to balance both hemispheres of the brain.
- Inhale through the left nostril, exhale through the right; then switch.

Candle Gazing (Trataka Meditation)

- Light a candle, sit in a dark room, and focus your gaze on the flame.

- This practice strengthens focus, clears mental fog, and activates the Third Eye Chakra.

Herbs & Crystals for Third Eye Activation

- Drink mugwort or blue lotus tea to enhance psychic clarity.
- Meditate with amethyst or lapis lazuli, which stimulate higher perception.

Meditation Techniques for Inner Vision

Meditation is one of the most powerful tools for awakening the Third Eye Chakra. It quiets the mind, heightens intuition, and expands consciousness.

Third Eye Activation Meditation

Step 1: Find Stillness

- Sit comfortably, spine straight, hands resting on your knees.
- Close your eyes and take deep, slow breaths.

Step 2: Focus on the Third Eye

- Bring awareness to the space between your eyebrows.
- Imagine a deep indigo light swirling in this area.

Step 3: Chant the Mantra "AUM"

- Inhale deeply, and on the exhale, chant "AUMMMMMM" .
- Feel the vibration activating your Third Eye Chakra.

Step 4: Visualize Inner Light

- Imagine a bright violet light expanding from your Third Eye, illuminating everything with wisdom.
- Feel your intuition awakening.

Step 5: Receive Inner Guidance

- Ask a question silently in your mind.
- Trust the first image, word, or feeling that arises.

Lucid Dreaming & Astral Projection

A powerful Third Eye Chakra enhances dream clarity, intuition, and spiritual vision.

Lucid Dreaming Practice:

- Before sleep, set an intention: "Tonight, I will be aware in my dreams."
- Keep a dream journal to record insights from the subconscious.

Astral Travel Visualization:

- Imagine your energy body floating above you while meditating.
- This practice strengthens your connection to higher dimensions.

Conclusion: Seeing Beyond the Illusion

When your Third Eye Chakra is open, you:

- Trust your intuition and make aligned decisions
- See the deeper meaning behind life's experiences
- Gain clarity and insight beyond logic
- Experience a heightened spiritual connection

"By activating this chakra, you awaken your inner wisdom and higher perception, allowing you to see beyond illusions and into the truth of existence."

In the next chapter, we will explore the Crown Chakra, the gateway to divine consciousness and spiritual connection. Get ready to elevate into higher realms of awareness and universal wisdom!

Chapter 8: The Crown Chakra – Connecting to Higher Consciousness

Introduction: The Gateway to Divine Awareness

The **Crown Chakra (Sahasrara)** is the highest energy center in the chakra system, located at the top of the head.

> *"It is the gateway to higher consciousness, spiritual awakening, and universal wisdom. The Sanskrit word Sahasrara means "thousand-petaled lotus," symbolizing the infinite expansion of spiritual awareness."*

When your Crown Chakra is open and balanced, you:

- Feel deeply connected to the universe and your higher self
- Experience inner peace, clarity, and divine trust
- Live with purpose and a sense of unity with all beings
- Receive intuitive insights and spiritual guidance effortlessly

However, when the Crown Chakra is blocked, you may experience:

- A sense of disconnection from life and purpose
- Mental exhaustion, lack of inspiration, or confusion about existence
- Rigid beliefs that limit spiritual growth

- Feeling isolated, lost, or without direction

This chapter will guide you in expanding your spiritual awareness, aligning with your higher self, and using meditation and energy practices to open the Crown Chakra.

- **Formation Period** : adulthood
- **Location**: The top area on the center of head, right on the crown
- **Color** : Purple
- **Element**: Light
- **Nature of energy**: Yang
- **Sound**: OM

Expanding Spiritual Awareness

A *balanced* Crown Chakra allows you *to move beyond the limitations of the ego-mind* and *into a state of universal consciousness*. This shift expands your awareness beyond the material world, helping you access higher wisdom, intuition, and deep inner peace.

Signs of Spiritual Expansion

- You feel more present and at peace, trusting life's flow
- You see beyond surface-level reality and recognize deeper truths
- Synchronicities and meaningful coincidences happen more often
- You experience deep gratitude and unconditional love for all beings

Practices to Expand Spiritual Awareness

Deep Reflection & Contemplation

- Ask yourself: "Who am I beyond my thoughts, emotions, and identity?"
- Reflect on your soul's purpose and how you can align with it.

Letting Go of Ego Attachment

- The ego creates separation and limitation.
- Practice observing your thoughts without attaching to them.
- Ask yourself: "Is this my soul's truth or my ego's fear?"

Connecting with Universal Energy

- Spend time in nature, absorbing the energy of the sun, sky, and earth.
- Visualize golden light flowing through your Crown Chakra, connecting you to the infinite universe.

Reading Spiritual Texts & Wisdom Teachings

- Explore teachings from Buddhism, Hinduism, Taoism, or other spiritual philosophies.
- Reflect on profound spiritual questions, such as "What is the nature of consciousness?"

Living in Alignment with Your Higher Self

Your higher self is the most authentic, wise, and spiritually connected version of you. It is free from fear, doubt, and limiting beliefs. Aligning with your higher self means living with clarity, purpose, and divine guidance.

Signs of Alignment with Your Higher Self

- You make choices based on love, wisdom, and intuition
- You trust the flow of life and surrender to divine timing
- You experience inner fulfillment rather than seeking external validation
- You feel guided by an inner knowing beyond logic

Practices to Align with Your Higher Self

Listening to Inner Guidance:

- Pay attention to intuitive nudges and messages from within.
- Trust the wisdom that arises in meditation, dreams, and moments of stillness.

Detaching from Material Illusions:

- Recognize that true fulfillment comes from within, not from status, wealth, or achievements.
- Shift your focus from external success to inner growth and service.

Living with Purpose:

- Ask: "How can I serve the world in a meaningful way?"
- Align your actions with your soul's calling and highest values.

Practicing Surrender & Trust:

- Release the need to control outcomes and trust that the universe has a divine plan.
- Instead of resisting change, embrace the unknown as part of your growth.

The Role of Meditation and Energy Transmission

Meditation is the key to unlocking the Crown Chakra. It helps quiet the mind, dissolve ego-based limitations, and create space for divine connection.

Crown Chakra Meditation: Opening to Universal Energy

Step 1: Find Stillness

- Sit comfortably, spine straight, hands resting on your knees.
- Close your eyes and take deep, slow breaths.

Step 2: Visualize a Violet or White Light

- Imagine a radiant violet or white light above your head.
- See this light entering your Crown Chakra, expanding your consciousness.

Step 3: Chant the Mantra "OM"

- Inhale deeply, then exhale with the sound "OMMMMMM."
- Feel the vibration awakening divine awareness.

Step 4: Dissolve into Pure Awareness

- Let go of thoughts and merge into a state of pure being.
- Rest in silence, feeling connected to all existence.

Energy Transmission & Divine Connection

The Crown Chakra allows you to receive high-frequency energy from the universe, divine beings, or enlightened teachers.

> *"Energy Healing & Reiki – Receiving healing energy transmissions can clear blockages and activate spiritual awareness.*
> *Silent Meditation Retreats – Extended silence deepens connection to higher states of consciousness.*
> *Prayer & Devotion – Surrendering to a higher power can create divine alignment."*

Conclusion: Becoming One with the Universe

When your Crown Chakra is open, you:

- Feel deeply connected to the universe and all life
- Trust divine guidance and live in flow with higher wisdom
- Experience peace, bliss, and a sense of purpose
- Recognize yourself as part of the infinite cosmic energy

> *"The journey of chakra mastery begins at the Root and ends at the Crown, but the transformation is continuous. By aligning all your chakras, you embody your highest potential and live a spiritually awakened life."*

In the next and final chapter, we will explore **how to integrate chakra healing into daily life** so you can maintain balance, alignment, and spiritual connection in every moment.

Chapter 9: The Energy Code in Daily Life

Introduction: Bringing Chakra Alignment into Everyday Living

Balancing and activating your chakras isn't just about meditation sessions or energy healing practices—it's about *how you live your day-to-day life.*

> "*The energy you cultivate through your thoughts, emotions, habits, and choices directly affects your chakras and overall well-being.*"

When your chakras are aligned, you:

- Feel physically, emotionally, and mentally balanced
- Experience clarity, inner peace, and purpose
- Attract positive experiences and relationships effortlessly
- Navigate challenges with ease and resilience

However, when your chakras are misaligned, you may:

- Feel emotionally drained or physically unwell
- Struggle with confusion, self-doubt, or lack of motivation
- Experience repeating negative patterns in relationships or work
- Feel disconnected from your higher self and intuition

In this chapter, we'll *explore practical ways* to *align your chakras through daily habits, create a high-frequency lifestyle, and establish simple chakra self-check practices.*

Aligning Chakras with Daily Habits

Each chakra governs different aspects of your life. By aligning daily habits with each chakra, you can cultivate balance and harmony.

Root Chakra (Muladhara) – Stability & Security

- Morning Grounding Practice – Walk barefoot on grass or earth for 5 minutes.
- Nourishing Foods – Eat root vegetables, proteins, and red-colored foods.
- Financial Awareness – Track your spending and practice gratitude for abundance.

Sacral Chakra (Svadhisthana) – Creativity & Emotion

- Creative Expression – Dance, paint, write, or engage in any form of self-expression.
- Hydration Ritual – Drink plenty of water to keep energy flowing.
- Emotional Release – Practice journaling or deep breathing when emotions arise.

Solar Plexus Chakra (Manipura) – Confidence & Power

- Morning Affirmations – Say "I am powerful, I trust myself, I take action."
- Physical Movement – Engage in core-strengthening exercises (yoga, pilates, or cardio).
- Decision-Making Practice – Make one empowered choice daily without hesitation.

Heart Chakra (Anahata) – Love & Compassion

- Self-Love Ritual – Look in the mirror and say "I love and accept myself completely."
- Acts of Kindness – Perform a small act of love for someone each day.
- Heart-Opening Exercises – Practice heart-opening yoga poses (e.g., camel pose, cobra pose).

Throat Chakra (Vishuddha) – Communication & Truth

- Mindful Speech – Before speaking, ask: "Is it true? Is it necessary? Is it kind?"
- Daily Vocal Exercise – Hum, chant, or sing to clear throat energy.
- Hydration – Drink warm herbal teas to soothe and open the throat chakra.

Third Eye Chakra (Ajna) – Intuition & Wisdom

- Daily Reflection – Spend 5 minutes in silence, observing thoughts without judgment.
- Dream Journal – Record dreams each morning to strengthen intuition and insight.
- Avoid Information Overload – Limit screen time and trust your inner guidance.

Crown Chakra (Sahasrara) – Spiritual Connection

- Morning Gratitude – Start your day by expressing gratitude for life.
- Meditation Practice – Spend 10 minutes in stillness, connecting to universal energy.

- High-Vibrational Input – Read spiritual texts, listen to uplifting music, or engage in sacred practices.

By weaving these simple but powerful habits into your daily life, you create an energy system that is strong, vibrant, and aligned.

Creating a High-Frequency Lifestyle

Your vibration—or energy frequency—determines the quality of your experiences. When your energy is high and balanced, you attract positive opportunities, relationships, and a sense of ease.

How to Raise Your Energy Frequency Daily

Nourish Your Body with High-Vibration Foods

- Eat fresh, organic, plant-based foods (fruits, vegetables, nuts, seeds).
- Avoid processed, artificial, and energy-draining foods.

Surround Yourself with High-Vibrational Sound

- Listen to healing music, mantras, or singing bowls.
- Avoid negative, chaotic noise or low-energy conversations.

Connect with Nature & Sunlight

- Spend time outdoors to recharge your aura.
- Expose yourself to natural sunlight for at least 10 minutes daily.

Practice Mindfulness & Gratitude

- Express gratitude daily—it instantly raises your vibration.
- Stay present, avoiding excessive worry about the past or future.

Choose Uplifting Relationships

- Surround yourself with positive, supportive people.
- Limit time with those who drain your energy or spread negativity.

Prioritize Rest & Rejuvenation

- Get quality sleep to allow your energy to reset.

- Engage in nightly wind-down rituals (gentle stretching, meditation, or journaling).

A high-frequency lifestyle isn't about perfection—it's about making small, intentional choices that support your well-being consistently.

Chakra Self-Check Practices

To maintain balanced energy, it's essential to check in with your chakras regularly. These simple self-check practices help identify and realign any imbalances before they manifest as physical or emotional distress.

Daily Chakra Self-Check

- Sit in stillness for 5 minutes and scan your body.
- Ask yourself: "Which chakra feels strong today? Which feels blocked?"
- Notice any tension, emotions, or energetic shifts in different areas of your body.
- Use affirmations, breathwork, or movement to support any chakra that feels misaligned.

Weekly Chakra Energy Audit

- Root Chakra – Do I feel grounded and secure this week?
- Sacral Chakra – Have I expressed creativity and allowed emotional flow?
- Solar Plexus Chakra – Did I take action toward my goals with confidence?
- Heart Chakra – Have I given and received love openly?
- Throat Chakra – Did I speak my truth with authenticity?
- Third Eye Chakra – Have I trusted my intuition and inner wisdom?
- Crown Chakra – Have I nurtured my spiritual connection?

If you feel imbalances, use the daily practices and chakra activation techniques shared in previous chapters to restore harmony.

Conclusion: Embodying the Energy Code

"Your chakras are living energy centers—not just concepts, but dynamic forces that shape your daily experience. By aligning your habits, raising your frequency, and practicing chakra self-checks, you create a balanced, vibrant, and purpose-driven life."

When your chakras are in harmony, you:

- Feel deeply connected to yourself and the universe
- Experience emotional stability, physical health, and mental clarity
- Manifest your highest potential with ease
- Navigate life with confidence, wisdom, and joy

"The journey of chakra mastery is not a destination but a lifelong practice. Each day, with every conscious choice, you are activating your energy, elevating your life, and stepping into your true power."

"You are the energy you cultivate. Live with intention, align with your highest self, and embrace the magic of your awakened energy."

CHAPTER ELEVEN

Chapter 10: Advanced Energy Mastery Practices

Introduction: Elevating Your Energy Mastery

By now, you have explored the *foundational practices of chakra alignment and energy activation*. In this chapter, we go deeper—beyond basic chakra balancing into *advanced techniques* that *amplify, sustain,* and *refine* your energetic mastery.

> "*Energy work is not just about healing; it's about evolution. The more refined your energy system, the more clarity, strength, and spiritual connection you cultivate. The practices shared here will help you:*"

- Expand your ability to sense and direct energy
- Deepen your meditation and breathwork for greater transformation
- Integrate movement and visualization for enhanced energy flow
- Maintain long-term energetic balance with advanced self-regulation techniques

If you are ready to elevate your practice and embody the highest version of yourself, let's dive in.

Deepening Your Connection with Energy Work

1. Cultivating Sensitivity to Energy

To master energy, you must first *enhance your awareness* of it. The more sensitive you become to energy, the more effectively you can channel, direct, and regulate it.

Practices to Increase Energy Sensitivity

Energy Field Awareness:

- Rub your palms together vigorously for 10 seconds, then hold them a few inches apart.
- Slowly bring them together and pull them apart. Feel the tingling or magnetic sensation between your hands.
- This is your energy field. Practice directing it inward (for self-healing) or outward (for manifestation).

Nature Energy Connection:

- Sit in nature, barefoot on the earth.
- Focus on the subtle vibrations of trees, water, wind, and sunlight.
- Breathe in the energy and visualize it merging with your own.

Energetic Seeing (Aura Training):

- Stare at your hand against a neutral background.
- Soften your gaze and observe the light glow (aura) around your fingers.
- Over time, this practice strengthens your ability to perceive auras and energy fields in people and spaces.

Combining Breathwork, Visualization, and Movement

Energy flows best when breath, intention, and movement work together. Here, we explore advanced techniques that synchronize these elements.

1. Breathwork for Energy Expansion

Chakra Breath Activation (5-10 minutes per session)

- Inhale deeply and visualize energy rising from your root chakra to your crown.
- Exhale slowly, feeling the energy radiate outward.
- With each breath, imagine the chakra glowing brighter and expanding.

Fire Breath for Energy Clearing (Kapalabhati – 2-3 minutes)

- Take a deep inhale, then exhale in short, sharp bursts through the nose.
- Focus on the rhythmic pumping of the lower abdomen.
- This technique clears stagnant energy, boosts vitality, and awakens personal power.

Wave Breath for Emotional Flow

- Breathe in a wave-like motion from your root chakra up to your heart.
- Feel the rise and fall of emotions as energy moves.
- Use this practice to release stored emotional blocks and restore balance.

2. Visualization for Energy Expansion

Spiral Energy Activation

- Close your eyes and visualize a spiral of light moving through your chakras.
- Imagine it expanding outward, connecting you to the universe.
- This practice accelerates energy circulation and spiritual activation.

Golden Light Shielding (For Protection & High Vibrations)

- Envision a golden sphere of light around your body.
- Feel this protective energy field strengthening with each breath.
- Use this technique daily to maintain energetic boundaries and high frequencies.

3. Energy Movement Practices

Qi Flow Activation (Energy Circulation)

- Stand with feet shoulder-width apart, arms relaxed.
- Imagine energy rising from the earth, circulating through your body.
- Move your hands in slow, circular motions, directing the energy flow.
- This is a powerful practice for maintaining vitality and fluid energy flow.

Chakra Dance & Shaking Therapy (Releasing Stagnant Energy)

- Play rhythmic music and move freely, focusing on each chakra's energy.
- Shake your body to release trapped emotions and stress.
- This liberates energy and restores natural alignment.

Sustaining Long-Term Energetic Balance

"Advanced energy mastery is not just about deep practices—it's about sustaining balance over time. Here's how you can keep your energy system resilient, vibrant, and aligned for life."

1. Regular Energy Audits

- Daily Check-In – Scan your body, noting where energy feels blocked or excessive.
- Weekly Chakra Alignment – Reflect on each chakra's state and adjust practices accordingly.
- Monthly Energy Detox – Use fasting, sound healing, or meditation to reset your system.

2. Strengthening Your Energy Field

- Energy Hygiene Practices – Regularly cleanse your aura with salt baths, smudging, or sound healing.
- Energetic Boundaries – Avoid environments or people that drain your energy.
- Mindful Consumption – Be intentional about the information, food, and experiences you absorb.

3. Mastering the Flow State (Living in Alignment with Energy Cycles)

- Recognize when your energy peaks and rests.
- Honor your natural rhythm—work when inspired, rest when needed.
- Cultivate presence, surrender, and trust in universal flow.

Conclusion: Becoming an Energy Master

True energy mastery isn't about rigid routines; it's about a *lifestyle of awareness, flow, and alignment.* When you integrate these advanced practices, you:

- Enhance your ability to direct and sustain energy
- Strengthen your connection to the universe and higher self
- Effortlessly maintain balance, even in challenging situations
- Unlock limitless potential for healing, manifestation, and spiritual growth

"*The Energy Code is no longer just a concept—it is a way of being.*"

You are now equipped with the tools to activate, expand, and master your energy at the highest level. Your journey does not end here—it evolves with every conscious breath, every aligned action, and every moment of deep presence.

"*You are the master of your energy. Own your power. Live your light.*"

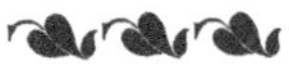

www.ingramcontent.com/pod-product-compliance
Lightning Source LLC
Chambersburg PA
CBHW040126150726
48005CB00015B/2392